Organic Coconut Oil, Apple Cider Vinegar, and Almond Oil Recipes

Disclaimer and Terms of Use:

Effort has been made to ensure that the information in this book is accurate and complete, however, the author and the publisher do not warrant the accuracy of the information, text and graphics contained within the book due to the rapidly changing nature of science, research, known and unknown facts and internet. The Author and the publisher do not hold any responsibility for errors, omissions or contrary interpretation of the subject matter herein. This book is presented solely for motivational and informational purposes only.

Table of Contents

Introduction

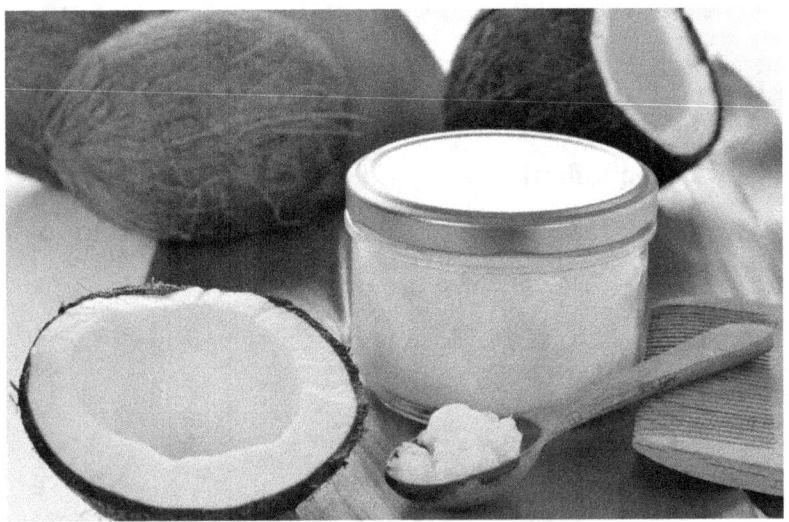

Even if you are not a health expert you have probably heard the term "superfood" tossed around. The term superfood is used to describe foods that offer significant health benefits or that provide certain benefits for specific diseases or conditions. There are many different superfoods out there but three of the top superfoods are coconut oil, apple cider vinegar, and almond oil. Coconut oil is rich in healthy saturated fats, especially lauric acid which helps to increase good cholesterol (HDL) levels while decreasing bad cholesterol (LDL) levels. Apple cider vinegar is particularly beneficial for diabetic individuals because it helps to control blood sugar levels – it also acts as a digestive aid, helping to support the healthy bacteria in your gut. Almond oil provides a number of health benefits for your skin, hair and nails – it also acts as a natural anti-inflammatory and antioxidant. If you are ready to experience the health benefits of coconut oil, apple cider vinegar, and almond oil this book is the perfect place to start. Simply pick a recipe and give it a try!

Coconut Oil, Almond Oil, and Apple Cider Vinegar Recipes

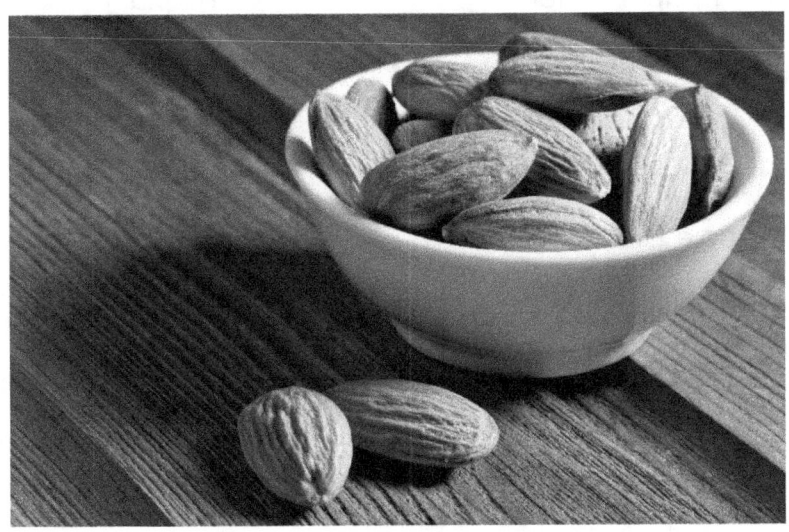

Recipes Included in this Book:

Crustless Vegetable Quiche

Almond Flour Blueberry Muffins

Tomato, Onion and Basil Omelet

Sautéed Sweet Potato Carrot Hash

Onion, Red Pepper and Spinach Frittata

Raspberry Coconut Muffins

Mushroom and Onion Omelet

Coconut Flour Chocolate Waffles

Cranberry Cinnamon Muffins

Sausage and Red Pepper Omelet

Cream of Broccoli Soup

Italian-Style Dressing

Apple Cider Vinegar Honey Tea

Lemon Cider Vinegar Dressing

Red Onion, Cucumber and Dill Salad

Curried Cream of Cauliflower Soup

Detox Hot Apple Cider

Cucumber, Tomato, Red Onion Salad

Almond-Crusted Baked Tilapia

Chocolate Almond Protein Smoothie

Skillet Steaks with Almond Oil

Tropical Mango Banana Smoothie

Coconut-Crusted Haddock Fillets

Almond Oil Hummus

Strawberry Coconut Almond Smoothie

Crustless Vegetable Quiche

Servings: 6 to 8

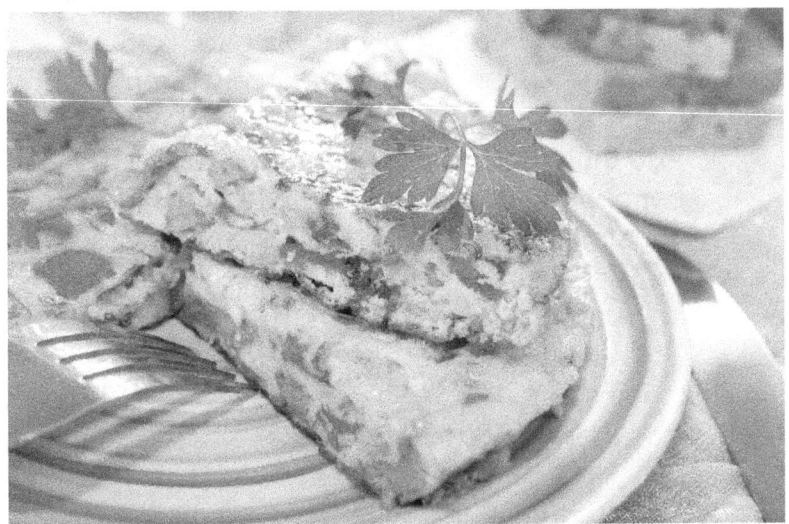

Ingredients:

1 coconut olive oil

1 medium yellow onion, chopped

1 cup tomatoes, diced

1 cup chopped zucchini

1 medium green pepper, cored and diced

10 large eggs, whisked well

3 tablespoons water

1 ½ tablespoon chopped chives

Salt and pepper to taste

1 ½ cups chopped spinach

Instructions:

1. Preheat the broiler in your oven to high heat.
2. Heat the coconut oil in a large cast-iron skillet over medium-high heat.
3. Add the onion, zucchini, tomatoes, and red pepper – cook for 5 to 6 minutes until the vegetables are tender.
4. Whisk together the eggs, water, chives, salt and pepper.
5. Pour the egg mixture into the skillet and stir in the spinach.
6. Cook for 4 to 6 minutes until the eggs begin to set.
7. Transfer the skillet to the oven and broil for 2 minutes or so until the eggs are set and the cheese is melted.

Almond Flour Blueberry Muffins

Servings: 12

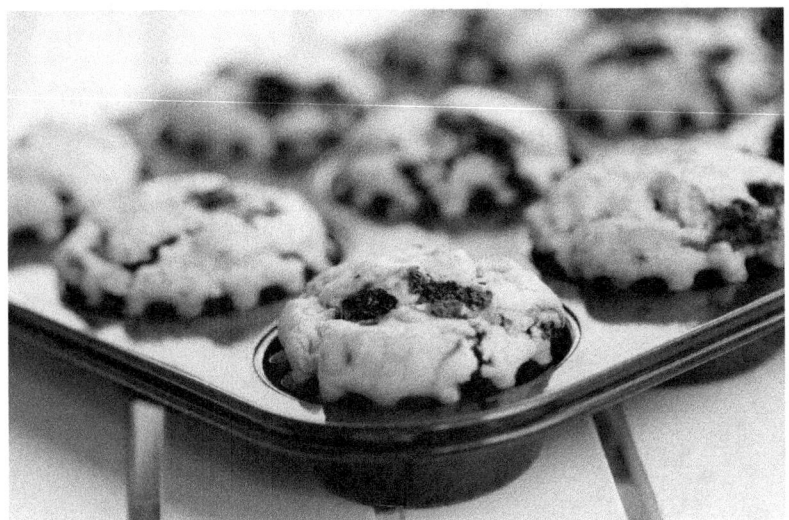

Ingredients:

2 ¼ cups almond flour

¾ teaspoon baking soda

¼ teaspoon salt

2 large eggs, beaten

1 cup unsweetened applesauce

5 tablespoons coconut oil, melted

¼ cup raw honey

1 ½ cups fresh blueberries

Instructions:

1. Preheat the oven to 350°F (175°C) and line a muffin pan with paper liners.
2. Combine the almond flour with the baking soda and salt in a mixing bowl.
3. In a separate bowl, whisk together the eggs, applesauce, coconut oil and maple syrup.
4. Whisk the dry ingredient into the wet until well combined then fold in the fresh blueberries.
5. Spoon the batter into the pan, filling the cups about ¾ full.
6. Bake for 20 to 25 minutes until a knife inserted in the center comes out clean.
7. Let the muffins cool for 5 minutes in the pan then turn out onto a wire rack to cool completely.

Tomato, Onion and Basil Omelet

Servings: 2

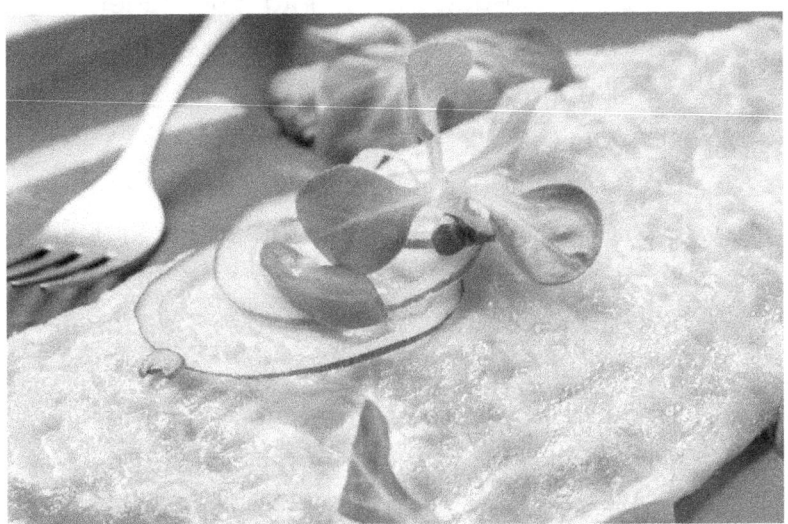

Ingredients:

4 teaspoons coconut oil, divided

1 large ripe tomato, chopped

¼ cup diced yellow onion

2 cloves garlic, minced

4 large eggs

1 ½ tablespoon chopped chives

Salt and pepper to taste

Instructions:

1. Heat 1 teaspoon of the oil in a small skillet over medium heat.

2. Add the tomato, onion, and garlic – cook for 3 to 4 minutes until tender.
3. Spoon the vegetables off into a bowl then reheat the skillet with the remaining oil.
4. Whisk together the egg, chives, salt and pepper.
5. Pour half the egg mixture into the skillet.
6. Cook for 2 minutes or until the egg is almost set.
7. Spoon half of the vegetables over half the omelet and sprinkle with basil.
8. Fold the empty half of the omelet over the filling and cook for another minute or until the egg is set.
9. Repeat with the remaining ingredients.

Sautéed Sweet Potato Carrot Hash

Servings: 6 to 8

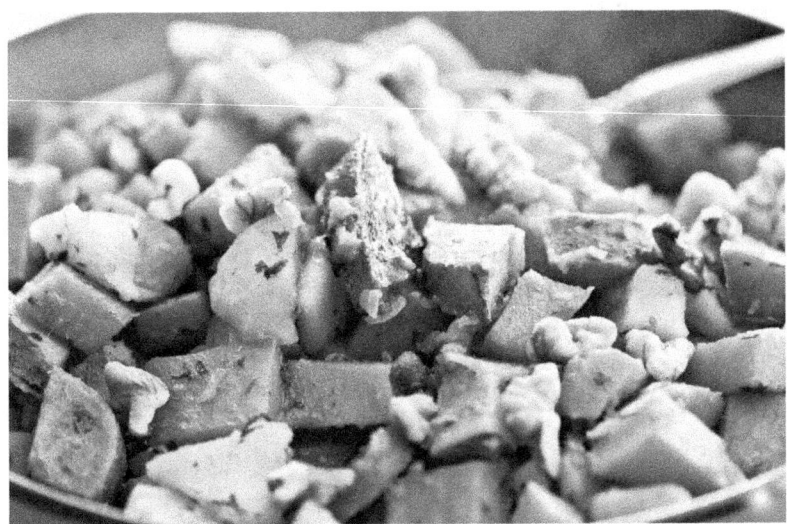

Ingredients:

2 tablespoons coconut oil

2 medium yellow onions, chopped

1 ½ cup chopped carrots

1 cup chopped cauliflower florets

2 large sweet potatoes, peeled and chopped

¼ cup fresh chopped parsley

¼ cup chopped walnuts

1 teaspoon chili powder

Salt and pepper to taste

Instructions:

1. Heat the coconut oil in a heavy skillet over medium-high heat.
2. Add the cauliflower, carrots, onions and sweet potato.
3. Sauté for 5 minutes, stirring often, until the onion is translucent.
4. Add 3 tablespoons water then cover and let the vegetables steam for about 2 to 3 minutes.
5. Remove the lid and stir in the parsley, walnuts, chili powder, salt and pepper.
6. Cook for another 4 to 5 minutes until tender and browned.

Onion, Red Pepper and Spinach Frittata

Servings: 6 to 8

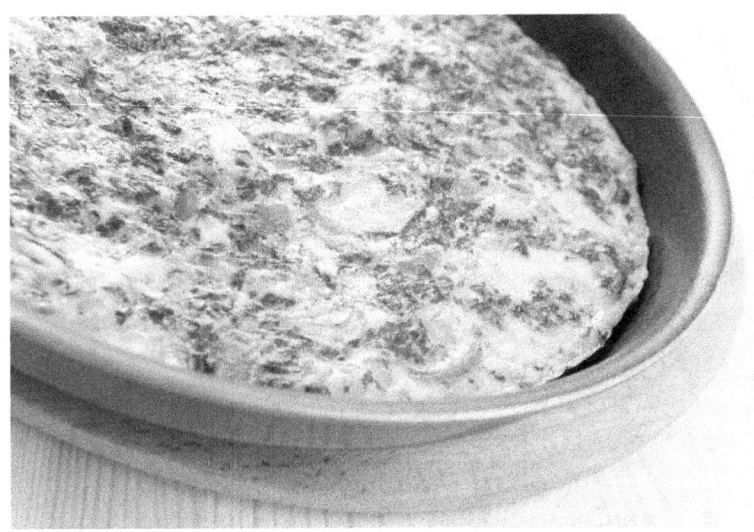

Ingredients:

1 coconut olive oil

1 medium yellow onion, chopped

1 cup zucchini, peeled and diced

1 medium red pepper, cored and diced

10 large eggs, whisked well

3 tablespoons water

1 ½ tablespoon chopped chives

Salt and pepper to taste

2 cups chopped spinach

½ cup reduced fat shredded cheddar cheese

Instructions:

8. Preheat the broiler in your oven to high heat.
9. Heat the coconut oil in a large cast-iron skillet over medium-high heat.
10. Add the onion, zucchini, and red pepper – cook for 5 to 6 minutes until the vegetables are tender.
11. Whisk together the eggs, water, chives, salt and pepper.
12. Pour the egg mixture into the skillet and stir in the spinach.
13. Cook for 4 to 6 minutes until the eggs begin to set then sprinkle with cheese.
14. Transfer the skillet to the oven and broil for 2 minutes or so until the eggs are set and the cheese is melted.

Raspberry Coconut Muffins

Servings: 12 to 14

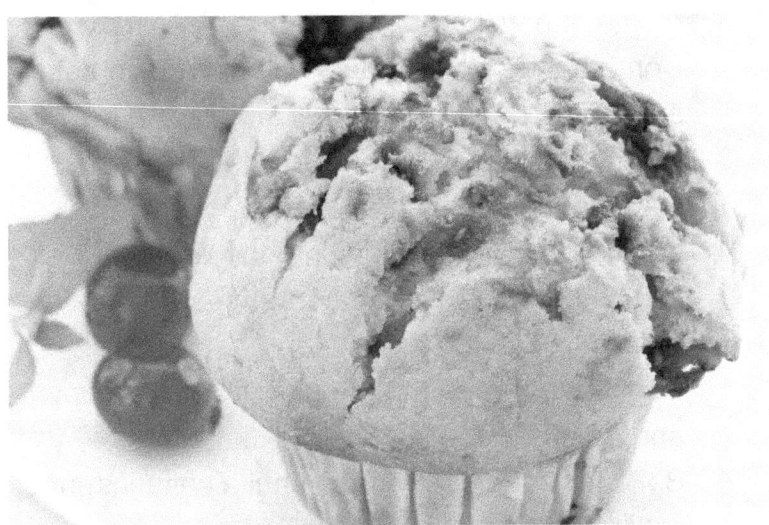

Ingredients:

2 ¼ cups almond flour

¾ teaspoon baking soda

¼ teaspoon salt

2 large eggs, beaten

1 cup unsweetened applesauce

5 tablespoons coconut oil, melted

¼ cup raw honey

1 ¼ cups fresh raspberries

½ cup shredded unsweetened coconut

Instructions:

1. Preheat the oven to 350°F (175°C) and line a muffin pan with paper liners.
2. Combine the almond flour with the baking soda and salt in a mixing bowl.
3. In a separate bowl, whisk together the eggs, applesauce, coconut oil, and maple syrup.
4. Whisk the dry ingredient into the wet until well combined then fold in the fresh raspberries and coconut.
5. Spoon the batter into the pan, filling the cups about ¾ full.
6. Bake for 20 to 25 minutes until a knife inserted in the center comes out clean.
7. Let the muffins cool for 5 minutes in the pan then turn out onto a wire rack to cool completely.

Mushroom and Onion Omelet

Servings: 2

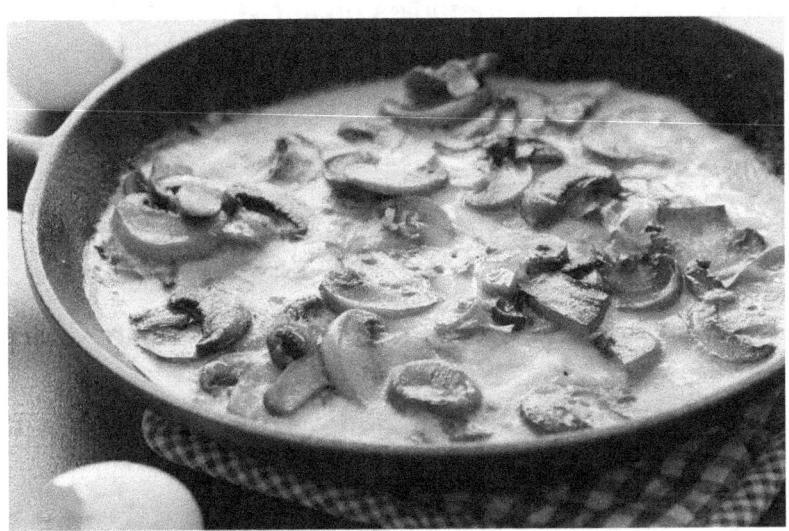

Ingredients:

4 teaspoons coconut oil, divided

1 cup diced mushrooms

¼ cup diced yellow onion

2 cloves garlic, minced

4 large eggs

2 green onions, sliced thin

Salt and pepper to taste

Instructions:

1. Heat 1 teaspoon of the oil in a small skillet over medium heat.

2. Add the mushroom, onion, and garlic – cook for 3 to 4 minutes until tender.
3. Spoon the vegetables off into a bowl then reheat the skillet with the remaining oil.
4. Whisk together the egg, green onion, salt and pepper.
5. Pour half the egg mixture into the skillet.
6. Cook for 2 minutes or until the egg is almost set.
7. Spoon half of the vegetables over half the omelet.
8. Fold the empty half of the omelet over the filling and cook for another minute or until the egg is set.
9. Repeat with the remaining ingredients.

Coconut Flour Chocolate Waffles

Servings: 6

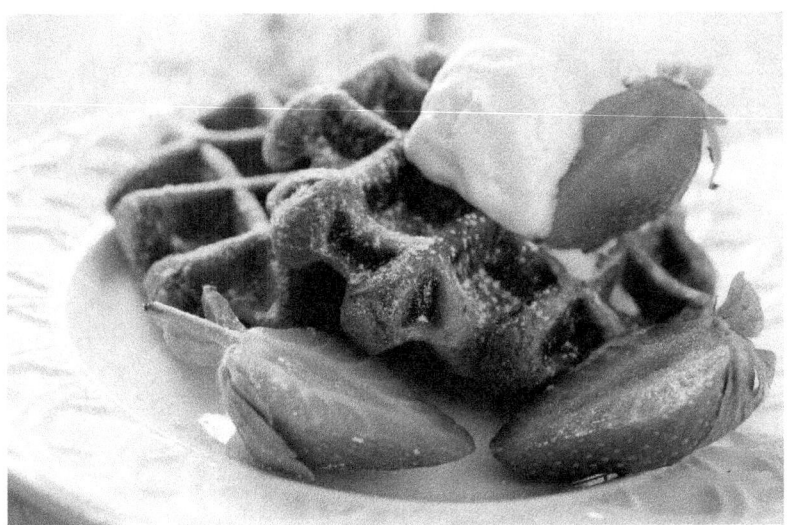

Ingredients:

6 tablespoons sifted coconut flour

6 tablespoons unsweetened cocoa powder

½ teaspoon baking soda

Pinch salt

4 large eggs, whisked

1/3 cup skim milk

3 tablespoons raw honey

3 tablespoons coconut oil

1 ½ teaspoon vanilla extract

Instructions:

1. Preheat your waffle iron according to the directions.
2. Combine the coconut flour, cocoa powder, baking soda and salt in a mixing bowl.
3. In a separate bowl, whisk together the eggs, milk, honey, coconut oil and vanilla extract.
4. Stir the dry ingredients into the wet until just combined.
5. Spoon the batter into the waffle iron and cook according to the directions.

Cranberry Cinnamon Muffins

Servings: 12 to 14

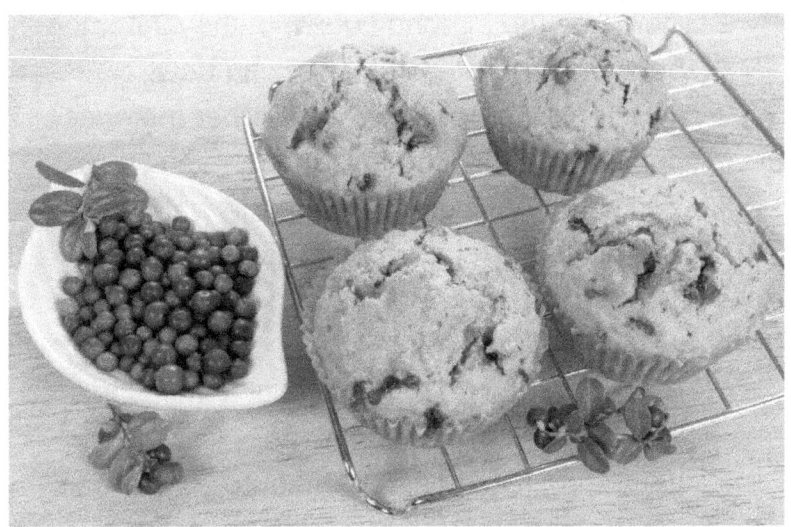

Ingredients:

2 ¼ cups almond flour

1 ½ teaspoon ground cinnamon

1 teaspoon baking soda

¼ teaspoon salt

2 large eggs, beaten

1 cup unsweetened applesauce

5 tablespoons coconut oil, melted

5 tablespoons maple syrup

1 ½ cups fresh cranberries

Instructions:

1. Preheat the oven to 350°F (175°C) and line a muffin pan with paper liners.
2. Combine the almond flour with the cinnamon, baking soda and salt in a mixing bowl.
3. In a separate bowl, whisk together the eggs, applesauce, coconut oil, and maple syrup.
4. Whisk the dry ingredient into the wet until well combined then fold in the fresh cranberries.
5. Spoon the batter into the pan, filling the cups about ¾ full.
6. Bake for 20 to 25 minutes until a knife inserted in the center comes out clean.
7. Let the muffins cool for 5 minutes in the pan then turn out onto a wire rack to cool completely.

Sausage and Red Pepper Omelet

Servings: 2

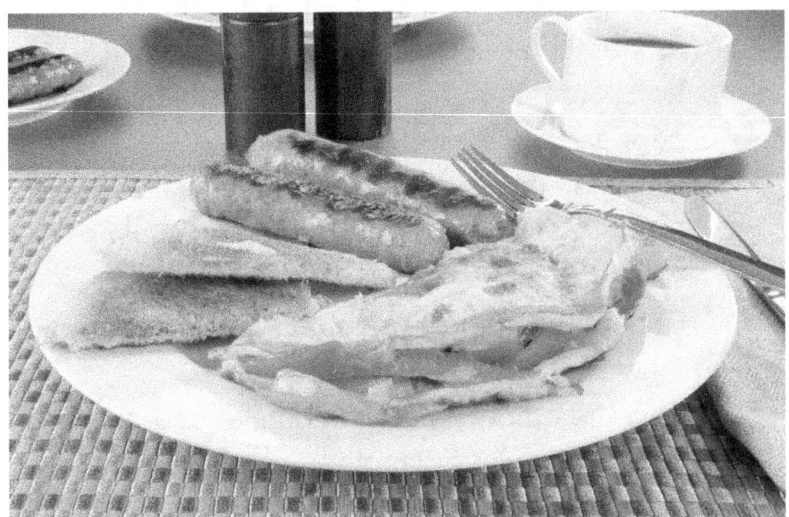

Ingredients:

4 teaspoons coconut oil, divided

1 medium red pepper, cored and chopped

2 links spicy sausage, chopped

2 cloves garlic, minced

4 large eggs

2 green onions, sliced thin

Salt and pepper to taste

Instructions:

1. Heat 1 teaspoon of the oil in a small skillet over medium heat.

2. Add the red pepper, sausage and garlic – cook for 3 to 4 minutes until the sausage is browned.
3. Spoon the vegetables off into a bowl then reheat the skillet with the remaining oil.
4. Whisk together the egg, green onion, salt and pepper.
5. Pour half the egg mixture into the skillet.
6. Cook for 2 minutes or until the egg is almost set.
7. Spoon half of the vegetables over half the omelet.
8. Fold the empty half of the omelet over the filling and cook for another minute or until the egg is set. Repeat with the remaining ingredients.

Cream of Broccoli Soup

Servings: 6 to 8

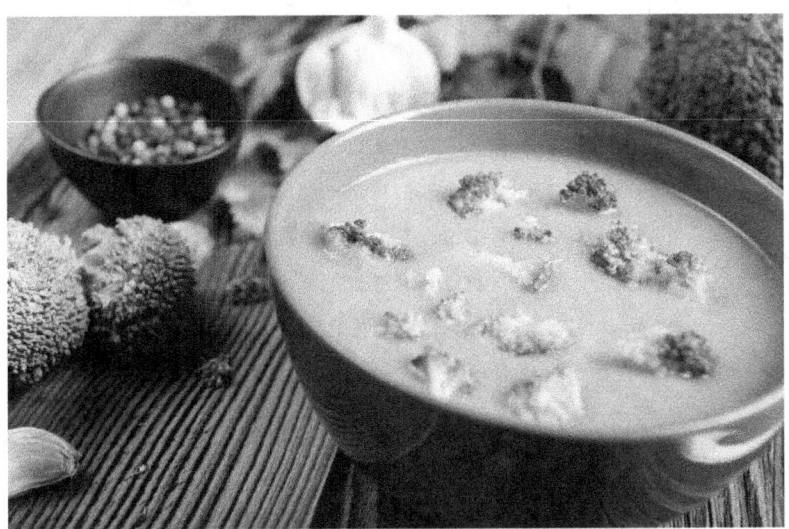

Ingredients:

2 tablespoons coconut oil

1 medium yellow onion, chopped

1 tablespoon garlic, minced

10 cups chopped broccoli florets

6 cups vegetable or chicken broth

1 to 1 ½ cups heavy cream

Salt and pepper to taste

Instructions:

1. Heat the coconut oil in a Dutch oven over medium-high heat.

2. Add the broccoli, onion, and garlic then cook for 6 to 8 minutes until tender.
3. Stir in the remaining ingredients except the cream and bring to boil.
4. Reduce heat and simmer for 20 to 25 minutes until the broccoli is tender.
5. Remove from heat then puree the soup using an immersion blender until smooth.
6. Whisk in the cream then season with salt and pepper to taste – serve hot.

Italian-Style Dressing

Servings: makes about ½ cup

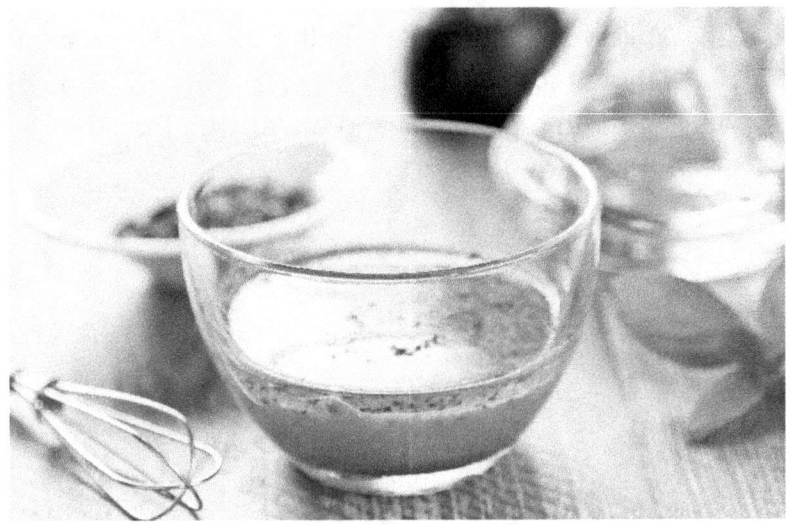

Ingredients:

½ cup extra-virgin olive oil

2 ½ tablespoons apple cider vinegar

2 ½ teaspoons coconut aminos

1 teaspoon ground flaxseed

6 to 8 drops liquid stevia

Salt and pepper to taste

1 clove garlic, minced

Pinch red pepper

Instructions:

1. Combine the apple cider vinegar, lemon juice, stevia and pepper in a bowl.
2. Whisk well until combined.
3. While whisking, drizzle in the olive oil – season with salt and pepper to taste.
4. Pour into a glass jar and cover with the lid – refrigerate.

Apple Cider Vinegar Honey Tea

Servings: 4

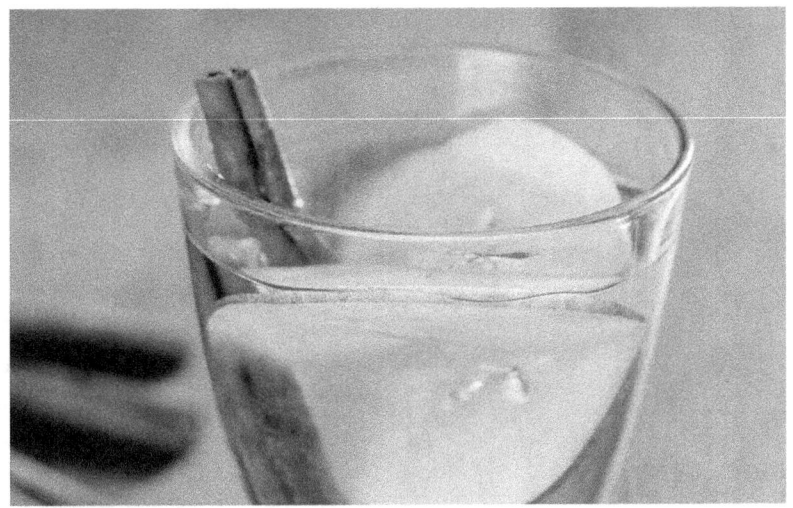

Ingredients:

4 cups water

1/3 cup apple cider vinegar

¼ cup fresh lemon juice

½ teaspoon ground cinnamon

Instructions:

1. Boil the water in a small saucepan.
2. Whisk in the honey, vinegar, lemon juice and cinnamon.
3. Divide among mugs and serve immediately.

Lemon Cider Vinegar Dressing

Servings: makes about 1 cup

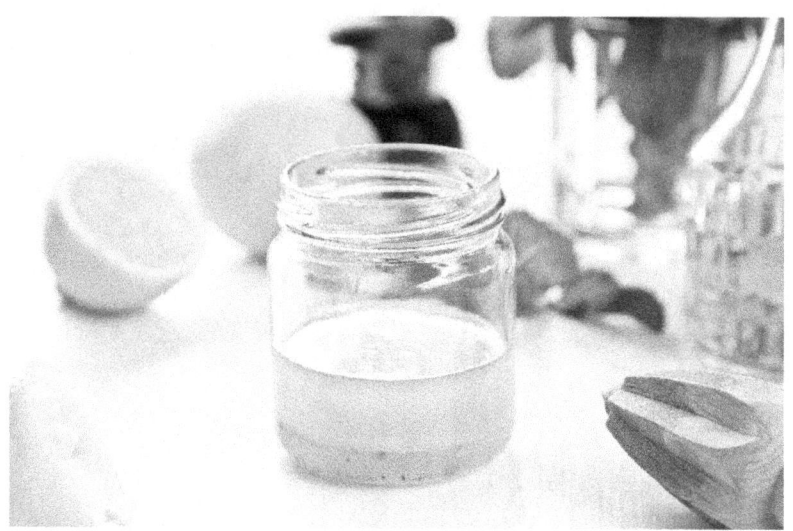

Ingredients:

½ cup apple cider vinegar

Juice from 2 lemons

1 teaspoon liquid Stevia

1 ½ teaspoons red pepper

½ cup extra-virgin olive oil

Salt and pepper to taste

Instructions:

1. Combine the apple cider vinegar, lemon juice, stevia and pepper in a bowl.
2. Whisk well until combined.

3. While whisking, drizzle in the olive oil – season with salt and pepper to taste.
4. Pour into a glass jar and cover with the lid – refrigerate.

Red Onion, Cucumber and Dill Salad

Servings: 6 to 8

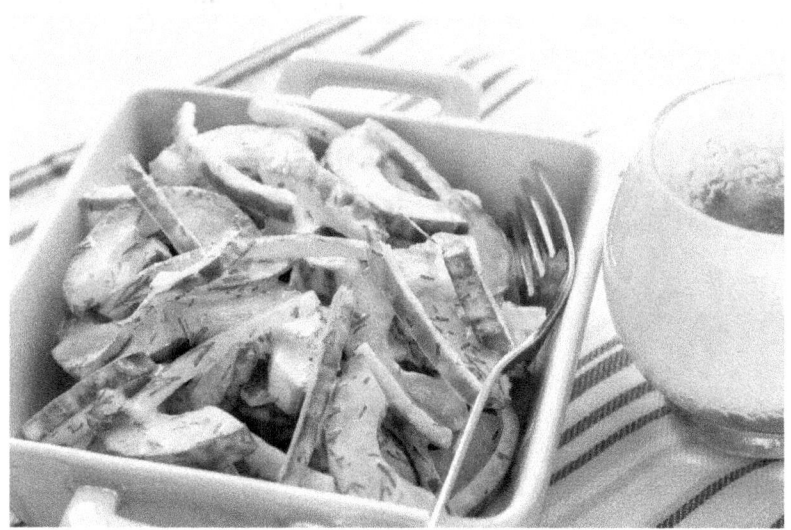

Ingredients:

2 ½ tablespoons apple cider vinegar

1 tablespoon raw honey

1 tablespoon Dijon mustard

1 ½ large English cucumber, sliced thin

1 small red onion, sliced thin

2 tablespoons chopped dill

Salt and pepper to taste

Instructions:

1. Combine the apple cider vinegar, Dijon mustard and honey in a small bowl – whisk smooth.
2. In a large bowl, toss together the red onion, cucumber, and dill.
3. Toss in the dressing and season with salt and pepper to taste.
4. Chill until ready to serve.

Curried Cream of Cauliflower Soup

Servings: 6 to 8

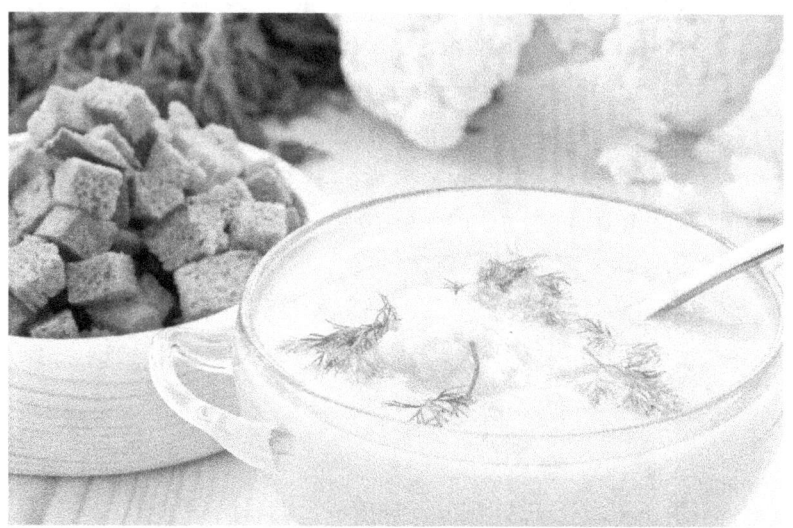

Ingredients:

2 tablespoons coconut oil

1 medium yellow onion, chopped

1 tablespoon garlic, minced

10 cups chopped cauliflower florets

6 cups vegetable or chicken broth

1 cup heavy cream

1 teaspoon curry powder

Salt and pepper to taste

Instructions:

1. Heat the coconut oil in a Dutch oven over medium-high heat.
2. Add the cauliflower, onion, and garlic then cook for 6 to 8 minutes until tender.
3. Stir in the remaining ingredients except the cream and bring to boil.
4. Reduce heat and simmer for 20 to 25 minutes until the cauliflower is tender.
5. Remove from heat then puree the soup using an immersion blender until smooth.
6. Whisk in the cream and curry powder then season with salt and pepper to taste – serve hot.

Detox Hot Apple Cider

Servings: 2

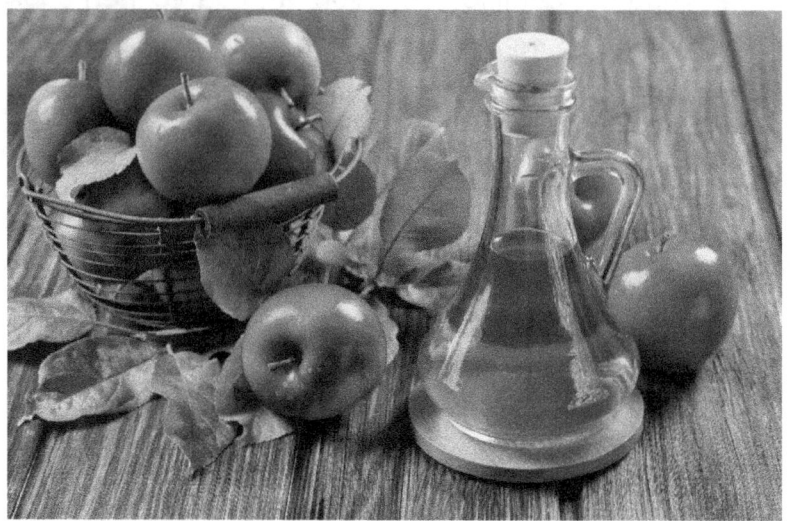

Ingredients:

½ cup water

½ cup apple cider vinegar

1 ½ to 2 tablespoons raw honey

1 teaspoon cayenne pepper

2 tablespoons lemon juice

Instructions:

1. Boil the water in a small saucepan.
2. Whisk in the remaining ingredients until combined.
3. Divide between two glasses and enjoy immediately.

Cucumber, Tomato, Red Onion Salad

Servings: 6 to 8

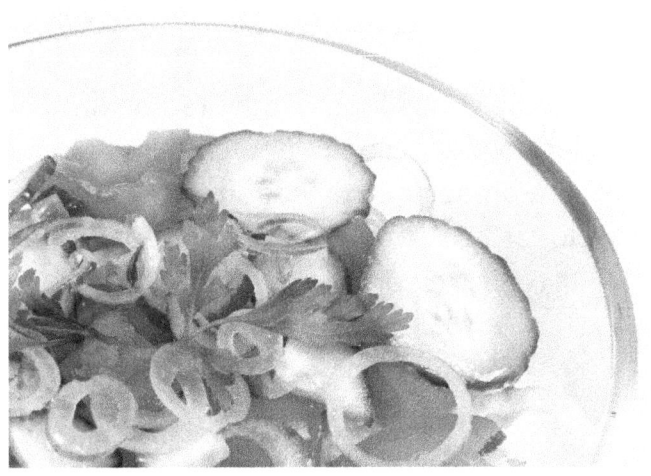

Ingredients:

2 ½ large seedless cucumber, sliced thin

4 medium tomatoes, chopped

1 small red onion, sliced thin

¼ cup fresh chopped parsley

¼ cup fresh chopped cilantro

¼ cup apple cider vinegar

2 tablespoons olive oil

1 to 2 tablespoons lemon juice

1 tablespoon raw honey

Salt and pepper to taste

Instructions:

1. Combine the apple cider vinegar, olive oil, lemon juice and honey in a small bowl – whisk smooth.
2. In a large bowl, toss together the red onion, cucumber, tomato, cilantro and parsley.
3. Toss in the dressing and season with salt and pepper to taste.
4. Chill until ready to serve.

Almond-Crusted Baked Tilapia

Servings: 6

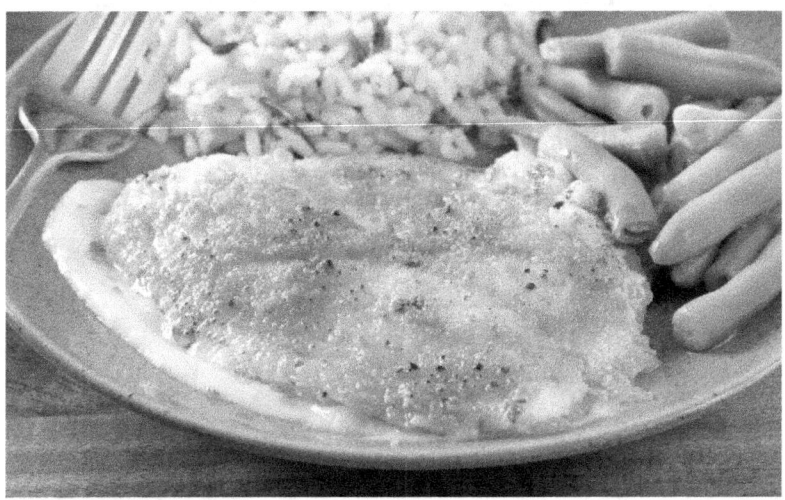

Ingredients:

6 (6-ounce) boneless tilapia fillets

2 to 3 tablespoons almond oil

Salt and pepper to taste

¾ cup grated parmesan cheese

1/3 cup whole-wheat flour

3 tablespoons finely chopped almonds

1 teaspoon dried parsley

Instructions:

1. Preheat the oven to 350°F (180°C) and line a baking sheet with foil or parchment paper.

2. Brush the fillets with almond oil and season with salt and pepper to taste.
3. Combine the flour, almonds, parmesan cheese and parsley in a shallow dish.
4. Arrange the fillets on the baking sheet and top with the parmesan mixture.
5. Bake for 12 to 15 minutes until the flesh flakes easily with a fork.

Chocolate Almond Protein Smoothie

Servings: 1

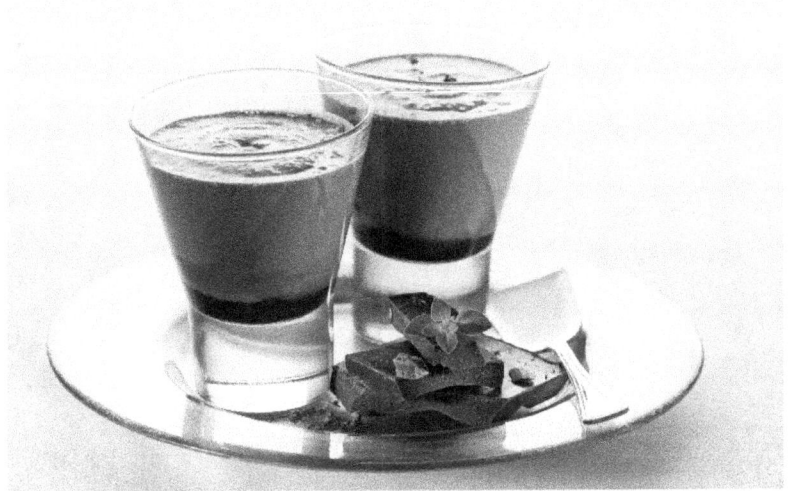

Ingredients:

1 cup plain Greek yogurt

½ cup skim milk

1 scoop chocolate protein powder

2 tablespoons chopped almonds

1 teaspoon almond oil

1 teaspoon raw honey

Instructions:

1. Combine the ingredients in a high-speed blender.

2. Blend on high speed for 30 to 60 seconds until smooth.
3. Pour into a glass and enjoy immediately.

Skillet Steaks with Almond Oil

Servings: 5 to 6

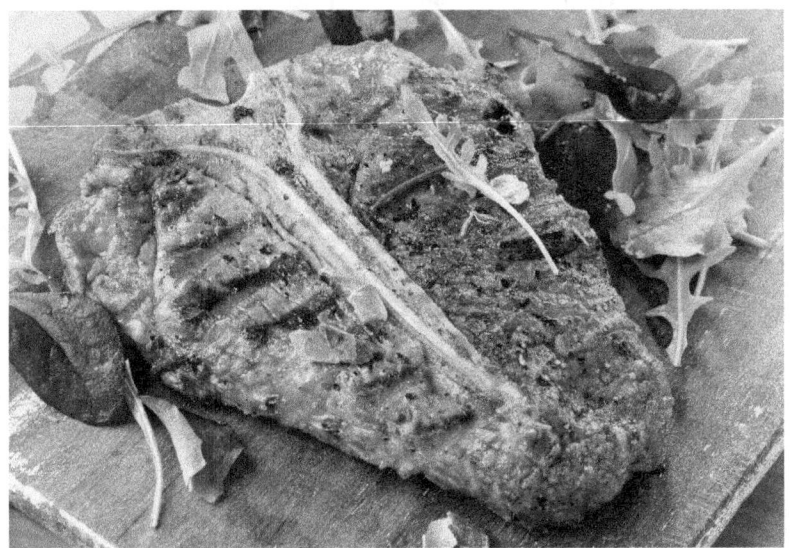

Ingredients:

2 (10 to 12-ounce) New York strip steaks

1 ½ tablespoons almond oil

Salt and pepper to taste

2 tablespoons unsalted butter

Instructions:

1. Heat the almond oil in a large cast-iron skillet over high heat.
2. Season the steaks with salt and pepper to taste.

3. Place the steaks to the skillet and cook for about 2 to 3 minutes on each side until browned.
4. Lower the heat to medium-low then add the butter to the skillet.
5. Cook for 1 to 2 minutes, basting the steaks with the butter.
6. Remove the steaks from the pan and place on a cutting board.
7. Cover the steaks with a tent of foil and let rest 10 minutes before serving.

Tropical Mango Banana Smoothie

Servings: 1

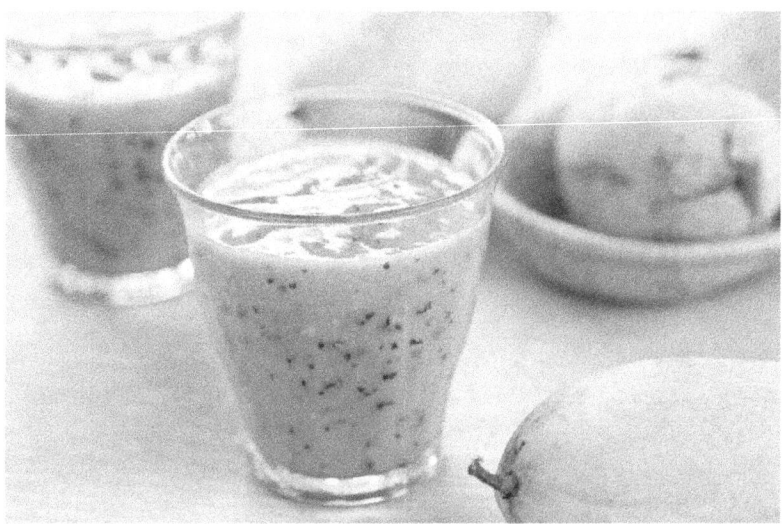

Ingredients:

Instructions:

1. Combine the ingredients in a high-speed blender.
2. Blend on high speed for 30 to 60 seconds until smooth.
3. Pour into a glass and enjoy immediately.

Coconut-Crusted Haddock Fillets

Servings: 4

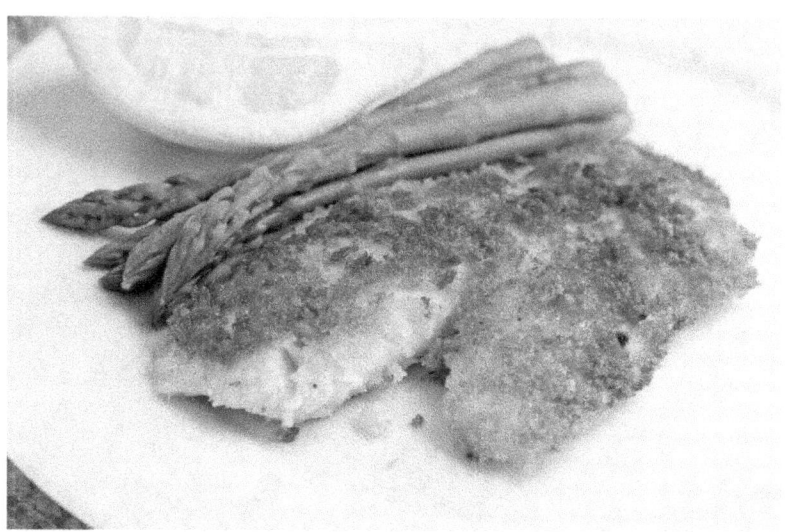

Ingredients:

4 (6-ounce) boneless tilapia fillets

2 tablespoons almond oil

Salt and pepper to taste

¼ cup whole-wheat flour

¼ cup unsweetened shredded coconut

2 tablespoons ground flaxseed

1 teaspoon dried parsley

Instructions:

1. Preheat the oven to 350°F (180°C) and line a
   baking sheet with foil or parchment paper.

2. Brush the fillets with almond oil and season with salt and pepper to taste.
3. Combine the flour, coconut, flaxseed and parsley in a shallow dish.
4. Arrange the fillets on the baking sheet and top with the parmesan mixture.
5. Bake for 12 to 15 minutes until the flesh flakes easily with a fork.

Almond Oil Hummus

Servings: yields about 4 cups

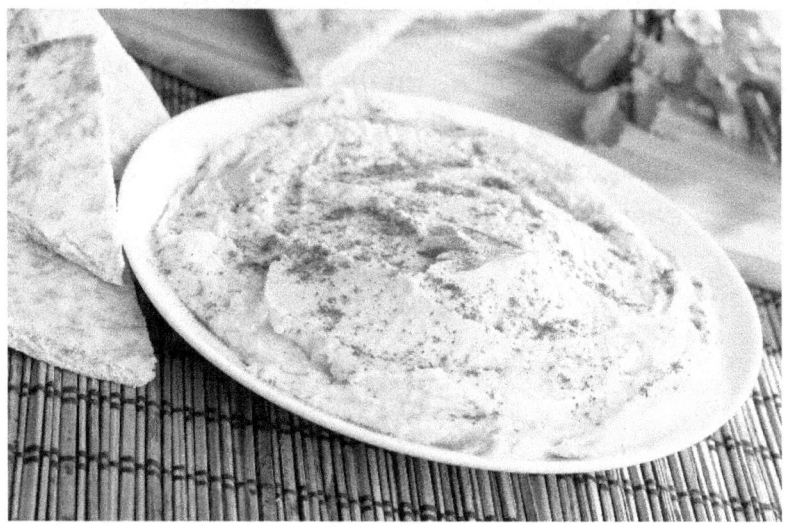

Ingredients:

2 ½ (15-ounce) cans chickpeas, rinsed and drained

¾ cups almond oil

2/3 cup tahini

½ cup plus up to 3 tablespoons water

1/3 cup fresh lemon juice

¼ cup chopped almonds

1 tablespoon minced garlic

1 teaspoon salt

Instructions:

1. Combine all of the ingredients in a food processor.
2. Blend until smooth and well combined.
3. Add a little more water or oil if the hummus is too thick.
4. Chill until ready to serve.

Strawberry Coconut Almond Smoothie

Servings: 1

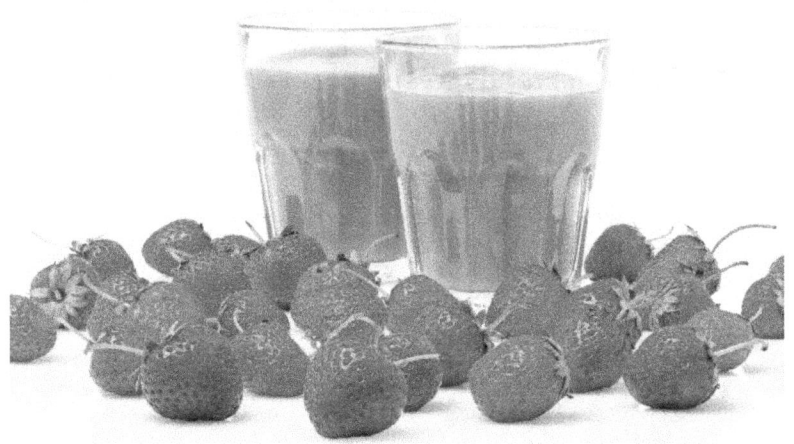

Ingredients:

1 ½ cups frozen sliced strawberries

½ small frozen banana, peeled and sliced

1 cup skim milk

½ cup plain Greek yogurt

2 tablespoons chopped almonds

1 teaspoon almond oil

Instructions:

1. Combine the ingredients in a high-speed blender.

2. Blend on high speed for 30 to 60 seconds until smooth.
3. Pour into a glass and enjoy immediately.

Conclusion

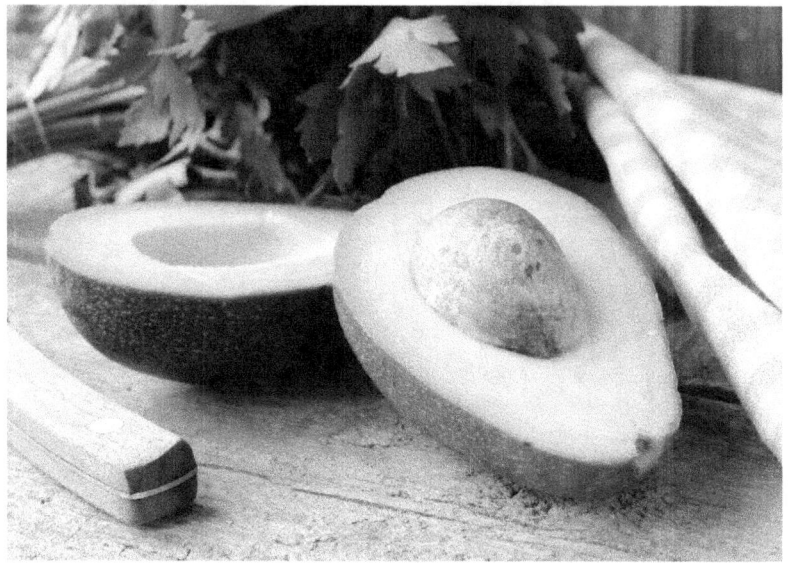

In some cases the term "superfood" is used rather loosely, but it is definitely well-used when it comes to coconut oil, apple cider vinegar and almond oil. These three foods each have their own unique set of benefits which can be used in combination to enjoy even greater benefits. If you are ready to experience the health benefits of coconut oil, apple cider vinegar, and almond oil this book is the perfect place to start. Simply pick a recipe and give it a try!

www.ingramcontent.com/pod-product-compliance
Lightning Source LLC
Chambersburg PA
CBHW070335290526
45791CB00003B/1334